AF866053

Welcome to My Practice—
Where Root Canals Aren't Scary Anymore

Sheila Chandrahasa, DMD

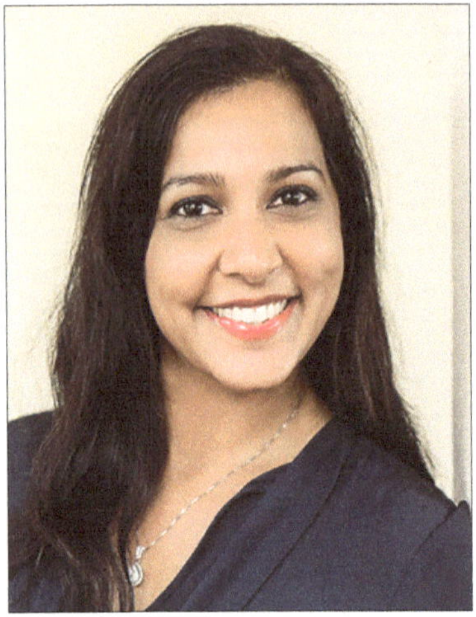

Sheila Chandrahasa
Doctor of Medical Dentistry

Why I love my work

I love having a practice where we quickly soothe and comfort nervous patients. Even though my patients are in pain and apprehensive when they walk into my office, they are smiling and laughing when they walk out.

Eliminating my patients' pain is the most satisfying component of my work. Seeing my patients happy again and knowing I was a part of that happiness makes what I do gratifying.

My ability to change the way people think about my profession is very valuable and is one of the reasons I am so passionate about educating people.

I hope this booklet will demystify root canal treatments and help many to realize the great importance of dental health to their overall health.

Dr. Sheila Chandrahasa

ISBN: 978-0-578-62609-3

© 2019 Sheila Chandrahasa
All rights reserved.

Contents

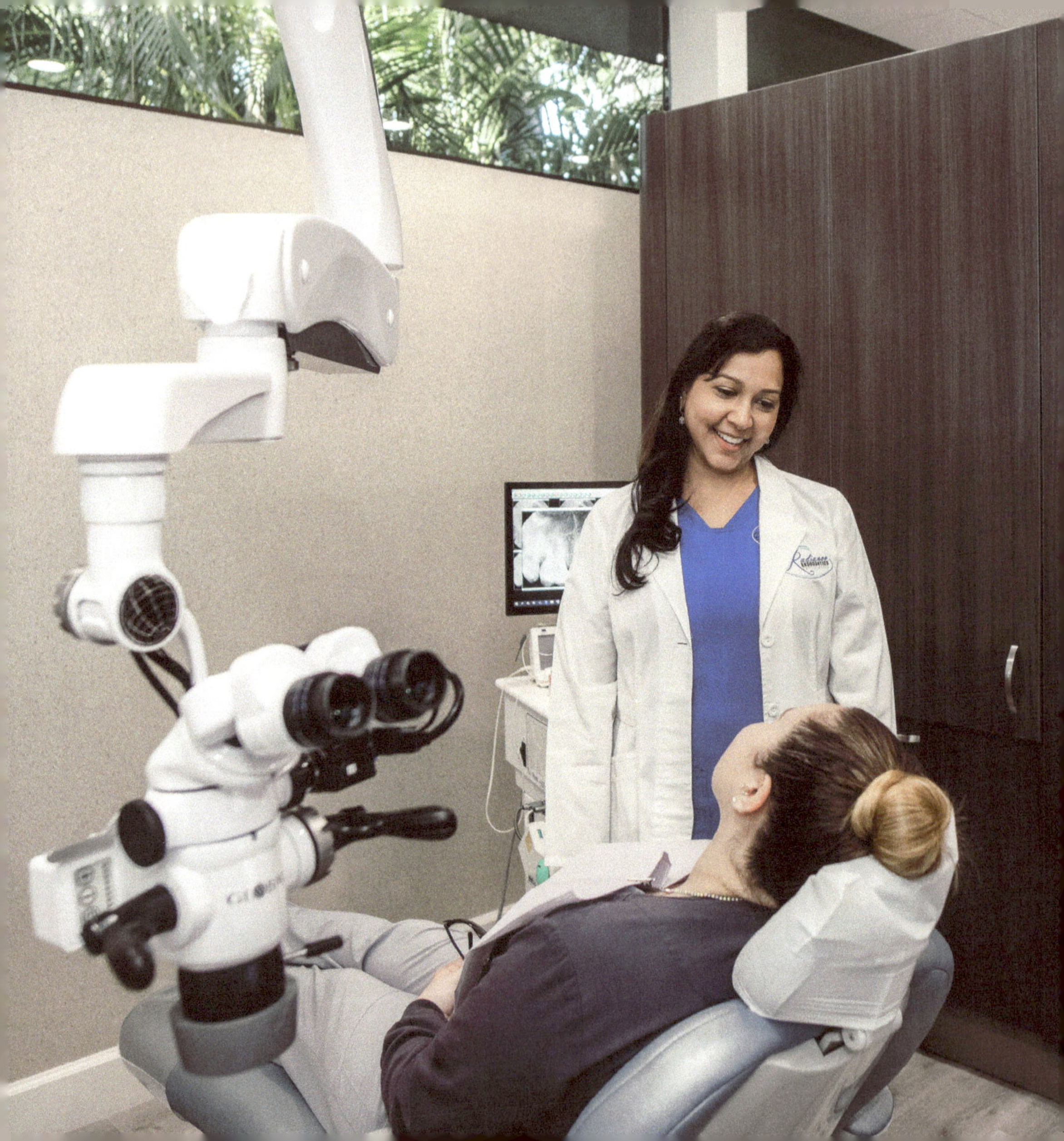

A toothache started my career in endodontics

It wasn't until I personally experienced a horrible toothache that I understood the difference between a dentist and an endodontist.

My toothache started after I had a really deep cavity filled; it was so deep that the filling was sitting on top of the nerve. The pain was so bad I couldn't eat or drink anything cold. And, of course, it was a Friday afternoon.

Fortunately, I found an endodontic resident who had a no-show on his schedule and he took care of me. A perk of being in dental school was I had access to many dentists and student dentists.

He numbed me up with some local anesthetic, placed the rubber dam and removed the tissue inside my inflamed tooth. Then he disinfected my tooth, sealed it with a temporary filling and sent me home with instructions to return in a few days to complete the root canal filling. That evening I had some discomfort, but took two ibuprofen and the next day I felt SO much better.

My endodontist was so kind, caring and compassionate that I started to think about how I could help people in similar pain—and that was the beginning of becoming an endodontist myself.

Principles that guide my practice

Patient health is #1

Healthy teeth are vital to your overall health and wellness.

Patient comfort is our goal

Relieving pain is second only to patient health.

Preserve the natural teeth

Natural teeth are designed for a lifetime; keeping what God gave you is in your best interests.

An informed patient is a happy patient

We want our patients to understand our diagnosis, recommendations for treatment and what to expect before, during and after the procedure.

What is an endodontist?

Endodontists are highly trained dentists who relieve tooth pain and strive to preserve your natural teeth. Endodontists are experts at root canal treatments. We are trained in the latest pain management techniques and in the use of specialized equipment designed for our profession, such as digital imaging and cone beam CT for diagnostics and an electronic apex locator and ultrasonic tools for the procedure.

Becoming an endodontist requires three to four years of dental school plus an endodontic residency program—an additional two or three years of education. This in-depth knowledge, training and specialized equipment make an endodontist the best choice for taking care of your teeth when there is an infection or injury.

Your general dentist and endodontist are partners

Think of your dentist like a general medical doctor and your endodontist as a specialist, like a cardiologist. You visit your general dentist for checkups and routine treatments, but they will send you to an endodontist to treat your special issues so you can have the best form of care. So, when problems arise involving your tooth's root canal system, your dentist will likely refer you to an endodontist, because we are experts in that area of dentistry.

Root canals demystified

The term *root canal* can be confusing because it is commonly used in two different ways. Let me clarify:

A root canal is a part of your tooth

The root canal is the natural tube located inside the root(s) of each tooth. The pulp is the nerve tissue and blood vessels inside each tooth that gives it life. Together, the root canal and the pulp is called the *root canal system*. (See the circled areas in the image on page 5.)

A root canal is also a dental procedure

A root canal is a dental treatment performed on an infected tooth to remove the infection, relieve the pain and save the tooth. We now call this treatment a *root canal treatment* or *root canal system cleaning*, which better describes the process.

During a root canal system cleaning, the endodontist or dentist removes the pulp, nerves and infected material from inside the root canal system and then disinfects and seals it.

Without treatment, the tissue surrounding the tooth will become infected and abscesses may form.

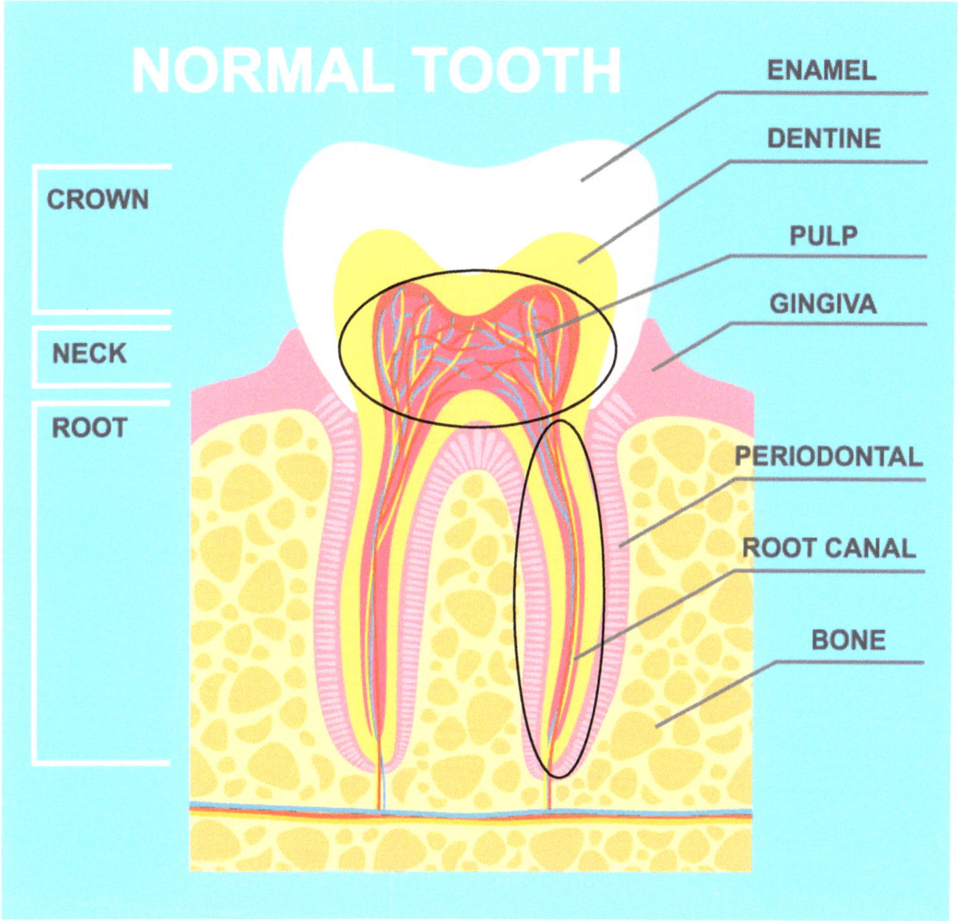
NORMAL TOOTH
ENAMEL
DENTINE
PULP
GINGIVA
PERIODONTAL
ROOT CANAL
BONE
CROWN
NECK
ROOT

Five ways endodontists increase success

1. Strive to preserve the natural tooth.
   It is in your best interests to keep your natural teeth. I strongly recommend a root canal system treatment to remove the infected tissue over removing the tooth, if possible.
2. Reduce patient pain during and after the procedure.
   Precise administration of local anesthetics manages pain during the procedure. Afterwards, over-the-counter pain relievers such as ibuprofen or Tylenol are usually adequate to manage post-procedure discomfort.
3. Detect the unique structure of every tooth.
   The specialized equipment in my office allows me to more accurately view the unique structure of every tooth. Though I usually describe the root canals as tubes, sometimes there are multiple tubes inside a single root.
4. Clean and disinfect the root canal system more completely.
   Because I am able to see the tooth's interior structure, I am able to clean and disinfect it more thoroughly, improving the success rate of every root canal treatment I perform.
5. Seal the root canal system with a bio-compatible filling material.
   The material used to seal the disinfected root canal system is *gutta purcha*, a natural, rubber-like substance from a tree.

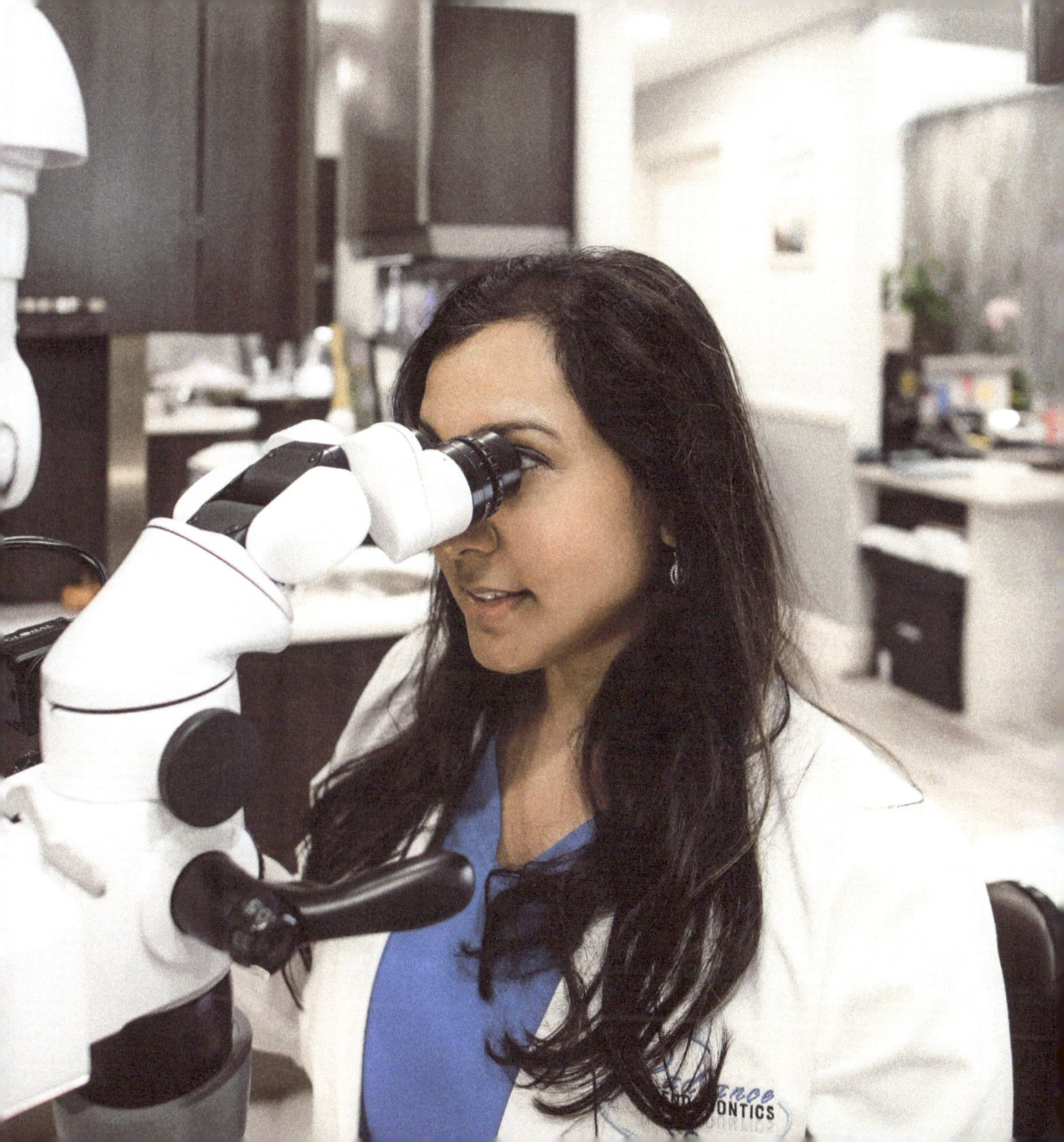

Why do I need a root canal treatment?

Once bacteria penetrates the nerve tissue inside your tooth, the entire root canal system will become infected. That infection will cause your body's immune system to react, which may cause sensitivity to cold or heat, swelling, inflammation and tooth pain. However, some people do not experience any of these symptoms.

The bacteria must be removed during a root canal system cleaning in order to eliminate the infection and restore health to the mouth.

Detect infection early with regular checkups

Some infections can lie dormant and you may not even know that the tooth infection exists. Then one day, you wake up with a swollen face.

Swelling may be one of the first indications of an infection. It's a red flag, signaling that your immune system is fighting a serious battle with bacteria and microorganisms. In extreme cases, these organisms can invade various facial planes in the head and neck that can lead to systemic illness. In the worst cases, these infections can block the airway.

These are important reasons why you want to get regular dental checkups and ensure any problems are fixed early.

Top 4 reasons you may need a root canal

The most common ways a tooth becomes vulnerable to bacteria and will likely need a root canal treatment are:

1. injury or trauma
2. fractures and cracks
3. deep decay
4. resorption

Top 4 reasons you may need a root canal

1. Injury or trauma to the tooth and tissues

Traumatic movement of your teeth and the ligaments that stabilize them creates a breach in the seal of the tooth, thus introducing bacteria into the root canal space. Trauma can also sever blood supply, causing tissue necrosis in the root canal space.

The American Dental Association reports that one-third of all dental injuries are sports-related, a compelling reason to wear a protective mouth guard when playing sports. Without the use of a mouth guard, risks are significant for injuries such as chipped or broken teeth, fractured crowns or bridgework, lip and cheek injuries, root damage and fractured jaws.

Children's teeth have the ability to recuperate from injury or insult due to the highly vascular nature of the root canal system and because the root ends of their teeth are not yet fully formed.

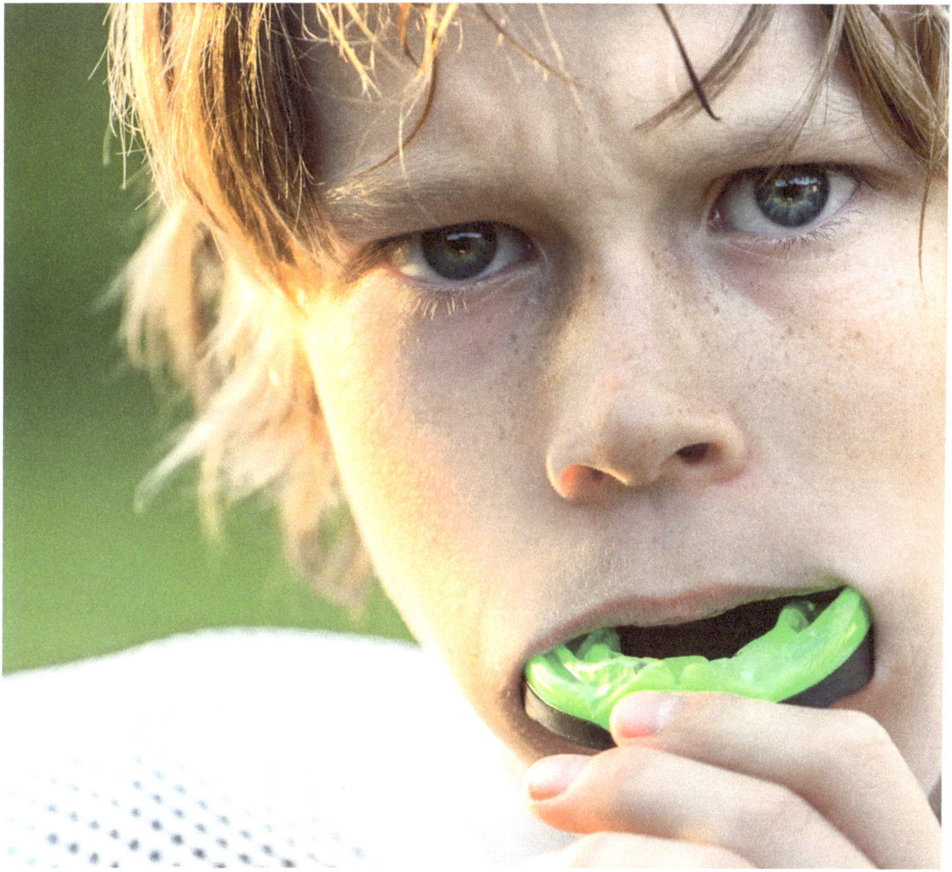

2. Fractures and cracks

Teeth will crack under pressure. When a portion of a tooth breaks off, the remaining tooth structure may be left weakened by micro-fractures. Those micro-fractures can allow bacteria to enter and infect the root canal system.

When the fracture is small and the fracture lines do not extend deep into the tooth or root, your endodontist will likely be able to preserve your tooth after a root canal system cleaning.

However, if the fracture is large and extends beneath the gumline to the root structure and deep into the tooth, it may need to be removed. Your endodontist will examine the tooth with a microscope to more precisely diagnose its condition.

Whether the fracture is large or small, a crown or cap will need to be applied to help dissipate the force of chewing and prevent additional breakdown of the tooth beneath it.

The most common causes of tooth fractures:

An imbalanced bite (occlusion)

It's physics: when you lose a tooth, the biting forces on the adjacent teeth increase. Conversely, forces dissipated over a greater surface area will reduce the stress and strain on each individual tooth. So, the more teeth you have to share the load, the better off you will be. This is why dentists will encourage you to replace missing teeth with a bridge, implant or partial denture to give you a more balanced bite.

Grinding (bruxism)

If you grind your teeth, you may want to speak with your general dentist about evaluating your bite and getting a custom night guard made for you. Night guards help protect your teeth by dissipating the force of the grinding across the night guard instead of directly on your teeth. In this way, it can help prevent future fractures and cracks.

Metal and large fillings

Amalgam can be an effective material to restore teeth but, because it is metal, it cannot flex like a natural tooth. This is why amalgam fillings or large fillings of any material may lead to fractures.

3. Deep decay

Cavities are a major cause of tooth infections and result from excess bacteria on the teeth. The acid produced by that bacteria erodes the tooth enamel and causes tooth decay. When tooth decay is allowed to continue without treatment, it can breach the sealed root canal system and infect the tooth.

Regular dental checkups and cleanings help prevent tooth decay. Periodic x-rays are also an essential diagnostic tool that detect tooth decay. Daily brushing and flossing are also essential to reduce the buildup of bacteria and plaque on your teeth and gums.

4. Resorption

Resorption is a destructive process—sometimes caused by trauma and tooth movement—that causes the tooth to eat away at itself. In some cases, root canal system cleaning can help stop the process of resorption by eliminating the tissue inside the tooth. If resorption progresses, the tooth may not be able to be preserved.

Regular checkups and x-rays with your general dentist may catch the resorption process early and halt its progress.

Stages and effects of tooth decay

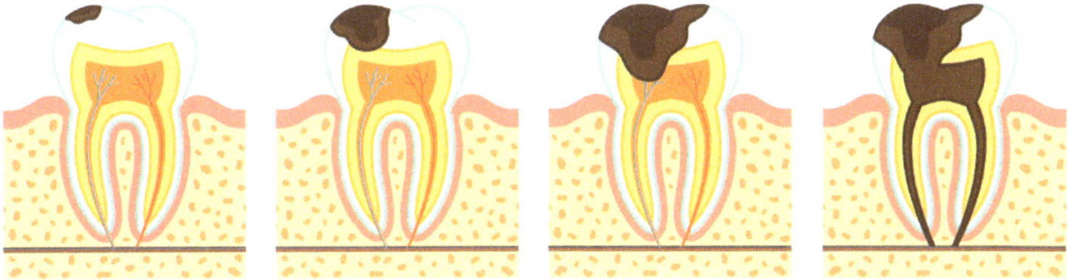

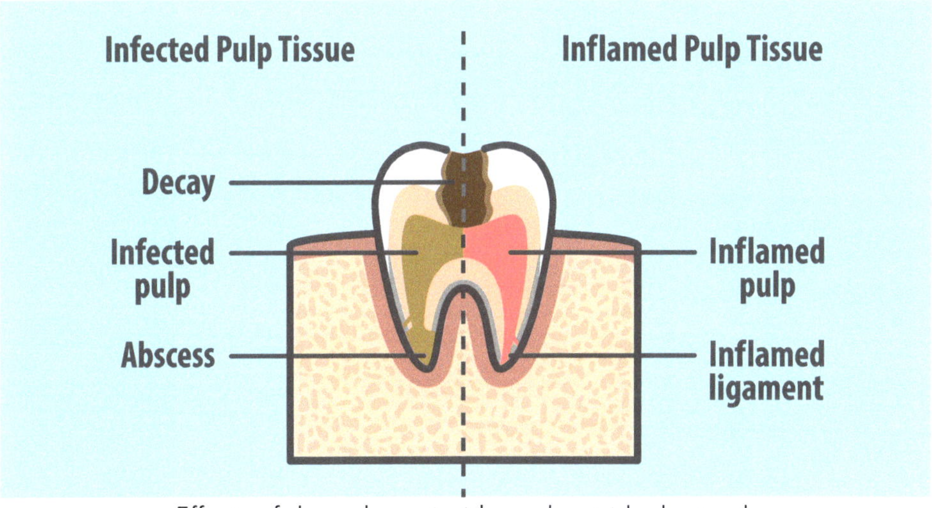

Effects of deep decay inside and outside the tooth

Myths and FAQs about root canal treatments

There are many myths about root canals that I'd like to clear up—an informed patient is a happy patient! The following are answers to the top questions my patients ask me.

Root canals are painful

Many root canals are essentially pain-free, others are uncomfortable. But your endodontist can make it nearly painless with anesthetic and a gentle procedure.

Every body is different, so everybody experiences pain in a different way. Some people have a higher pain tolerance, some have a lower pain threshhold. Patients who have a severe toothache before a root canal procedure often have discomfort after the procedure because a highly inflamed tooth or a significant infection takes time to settle down.

Some neurological conditions can mimic a toothache. Patients with certain neurological conditions may also have an altered perception of pain. An endodontist can help clearly diagnose if the pain is truly coming from a tooth.

Why can't I just take an antibiotic for the infection?

A dental infection is very different than, let's say, a bladder infection. Antibiotics go through the body to the site of the infection and are able to kill the bacteria because the source of the bacteria is generally external to the body.

A dental infection is very different because the bacteria is inside the tooth. Taking antibiotics for a dental infection will only suppress the symptoms; it will not eliminate the source of the infection because the source is the tooth. The two primary ways to remove a dental infection are a root canal system treatment or removing the tooth.

Why do I still have pain after the procedure?

Post-operative discomfort is very common because the ligaments around the tooth are alive and need time to settle down. Over-the-counter pain medications are generally adequate for this type of post-procedure discomfort. Your dentist may also prescribe an antibiotic for the infection to help the body heal.

Myths and FAQs about root canal treatments

Do I still need to take Advil or Tylenol if I'm not having pain?

We recommend that you take analgesics for three days after the procedure so they are in your system if pain occurs, which sometimes happens from 24 to 72 hours after the procedure.

Why can't I use a hot or cold compress after a root canal?

We don't recommend using cold compresses because the cold temperature may reduce blood flow and slow the healing process. At times, we may recommend a hot compress in cases of infection and swelling.

Will a root canal remove the actual roots of my tooth?

The misconception is in the terminology itself. The true definition of a root canal treatment is cleaning out the root canal system which consists of blood and nerve tissue inside the tooth. We are not removing the physical roots of the tooth; the roots remain intact in the jaw bone.

Why do some people need a second root canal?

A revision of an old root canal may be necessary for these reasons:

- Inadequate original treatment.
- Missed canal—Every tooth has a unique root structure; some may be difficult to detect.

- Bacteria or microorganisms not completely removed due to complex internal anatomy of the tooth.
- Root canals were not sealed correctly—The root canal system must be sealed from the crown to the root tips to prevent bacteria from entering the space again.
- Bacteria reintroduced due to a leaking crown or filling, cavity, grinding, occlusal trauma (biting down hard) or trauma to the tooth.

What is root end surgery?

When there is bone loss around the roots of a tooth, the area is filled with soft tissue and fluid. A pimple on the gum may appear to indicate a tooth infection. If bone doesn't get redeposited and the tissue becomes an obstruction to healing, you may risk losing the tooth. Alternately, your dentist may recommend an additional procedure called *apicoectomy*, or root end surgery. In this procedure, the tip of the root is cut off and the root end is filled with another type of special material. The area of the bone infection is also cleaned out.

I have concerns about radiation. Do I need x-rays?

X-rays are essential to help the dentist to see and diagnose conditions that are impossible to see with the naked eye. Your endodontist will take multiple x-rays from different angles and test your teeth to accurately diagnose if a root canal system treatment is necessary.

The benefits of having x-rays far outweigh the risks. Most dental offices now have digital x-rays which use a very narrow spectrum of rays to minimize radiation.

What type of material is used to fill the root canal space?

The root canal system is filled with a material that is compatible with the body but also easy to remove, just in case there's a problem and the root canal treatment needs to be revised.

What patients say about Dr. Chandrahasa and her staff

Well done. Very gentle-no discomfort. Always taking care of me, the patient. Painless. A good dentist experience!!!

R. Vanyo

Very gentle and caring during a stressful procedure.

S. Murdock

Very professional. No pain. Concern for comfort. Informative of every step. Courteous and prompt. Appointments on time.

G. Tucker

Step by step through a root canal treatment

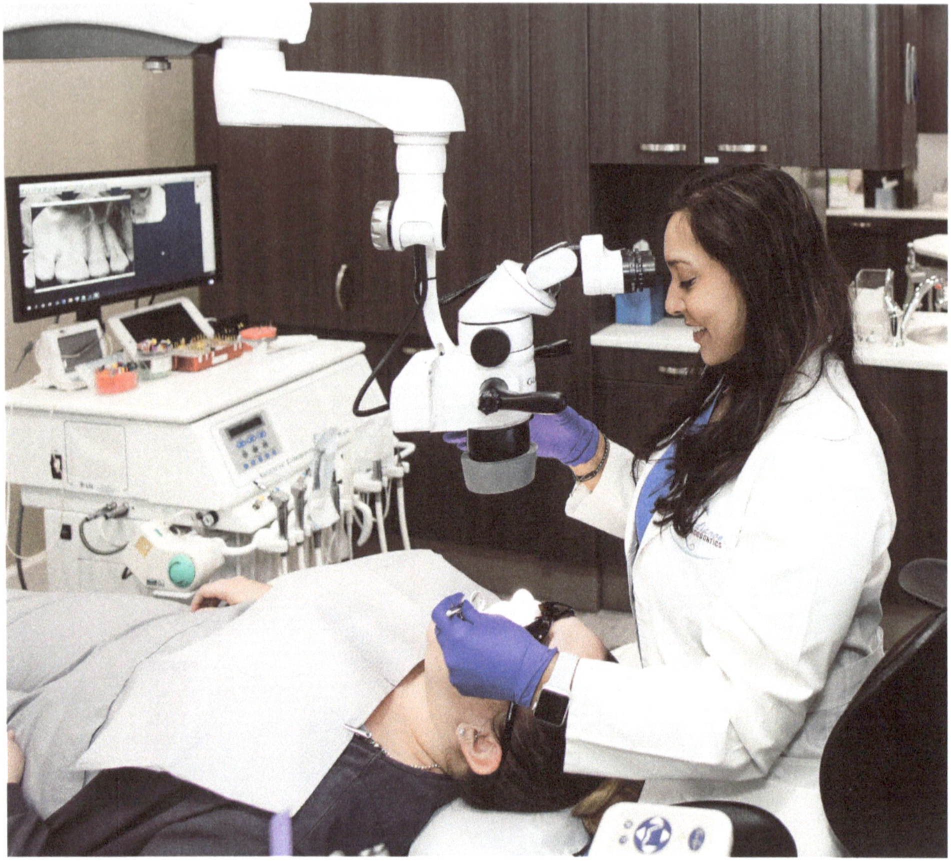

1. Anesthesia

Once a specific tooth is diagnosed, the endodontist will use local anesthetics to make you feel comfortable during the procedure. The goal is for you to not feel any sensation.

Many times, we're able to do a root canal system cleaning without pain, but there can be circumstances in which your tooth and the surrounding tissues are so inflamed you may have a hard time getting numb. Also, certain fibers inside the tooth may feel pain, even though the infected tooth and nerves may be dead.

In these situations, taking analgesics and various injection techniques may help alleviate discomfort during the procedure.

2. Rubber dam

At the beginning of the procedure, your endodontist or dentist will place a rubber dam around the tooth to be treated. This is a special shield used during a root canal system cleaning as a standard of care and is for the patient's safety. The rubber dam serves as a protective barrier to prevent the patient from swallowing or aspirating any of the small instruments used during the root canal procedure. Root canal treatments should not be done without the use of a rubber dam.

Step by step through a root canal treatment

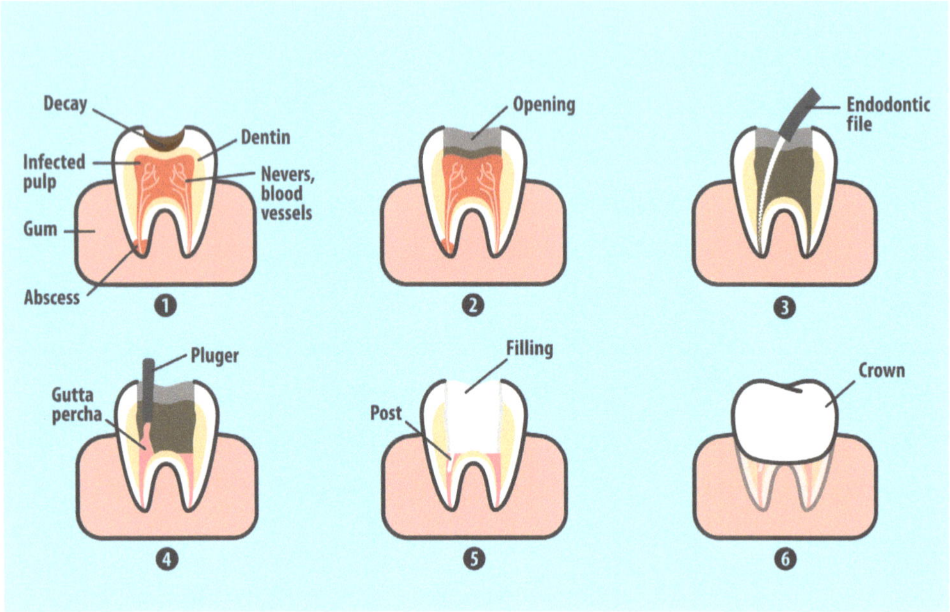

3. Diagnostic imaging

Your endodontist will use a microscope, ultrasonic techniques and may take special x-rays or use special imaging techniques such as the cone beam CT to better understand your tooth's anatomy, thus ensuring as complete a cleaning as possible.

4. Root canal system cleaning and disinfection

Various disinfectant solutions are used during the procedure to eliminate tissue inside the root canal system. Instruments are used to scrape the walls of the tooth structure to aid in debris removal.

5. Sealing the root canal system

Ensuring a complete seal of the root canal system is essential for sealing out bacteria. Various materials are used to seal the root canal space; some are heat-sealed inside the tooth.

6. After the procedure

Typically, your endodontist will place a temporary filling in the tooth to close off the tooth's interior. Your general dentist will place a permanent filling or crown as a last step.

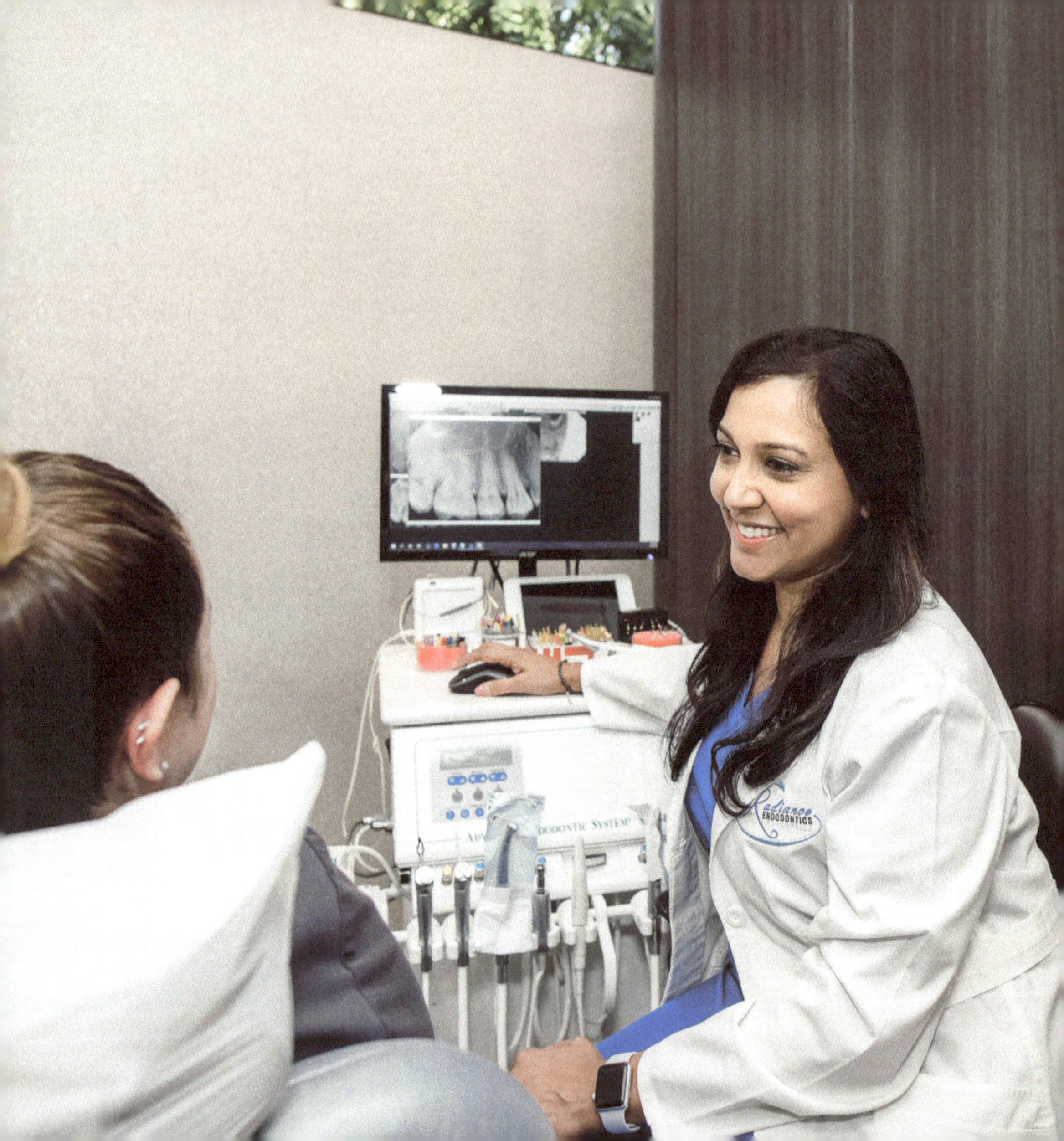
Radiance
ENDODONTICS

Healthy teeth = healthy body

There is great value in saving your natural teeth

Most of us value our teeth because a bright smile is attractive and we want to look our best. But many don't realize the importance of their teeth to their overall health and wellness. Teeth are essential for good digestion, help support your facial structure, lips, cheeks and help your smile.

What is unique to the natural dentition? Just like a hip or knee joint, each tooth has a joint supported by a periodontal ligament. The periodontal ligament helps cushion the forces on your teeth as you chew and function on them over time.

Preserving your teeth also helps you maintain the amount of bone mass in your jaw; the moment you lose a tooth, the bone in that area begins to melt away, which will affect the adjacent teeth.

The more teeth you have, the more balanced your bite will be. If you have to lose a tooth, it's best to replace it so your bite can be balanced.

Healthy teeth = healthy body

Healthy teeth are required for healthy digestion

Your teeth were designed to withstand a lifetime of chewing and to play their essential role in digestion. Digestion begins in the mouth where the act of chewing and the enzymes in saliva break down the food so it can be swallowed. Keeping your teeth healthy means a lifetime of healthy digestion.

Healthy gums help avoid root canals

If you have bleeding gums, please go to your dentist for a checkup and learn what you can do to improve the health of your gums. Healthy gums reduce the likelihood that you'll need a root canal system cleaning and risk losing a tooth.

Periodontal disease or gum disease starts a chain reaction that may lead to serious dental infections. At first, the gumline recedes, exposing more and more of the tooth root. When the root is exposed to the acids in food and beverages, plaque and bacteria will accumulate, causing bone loss. In addition, less supporting bone weakens the tooth structure and increases the likelihood of a tooth becoming infected.

Stages of gum disease

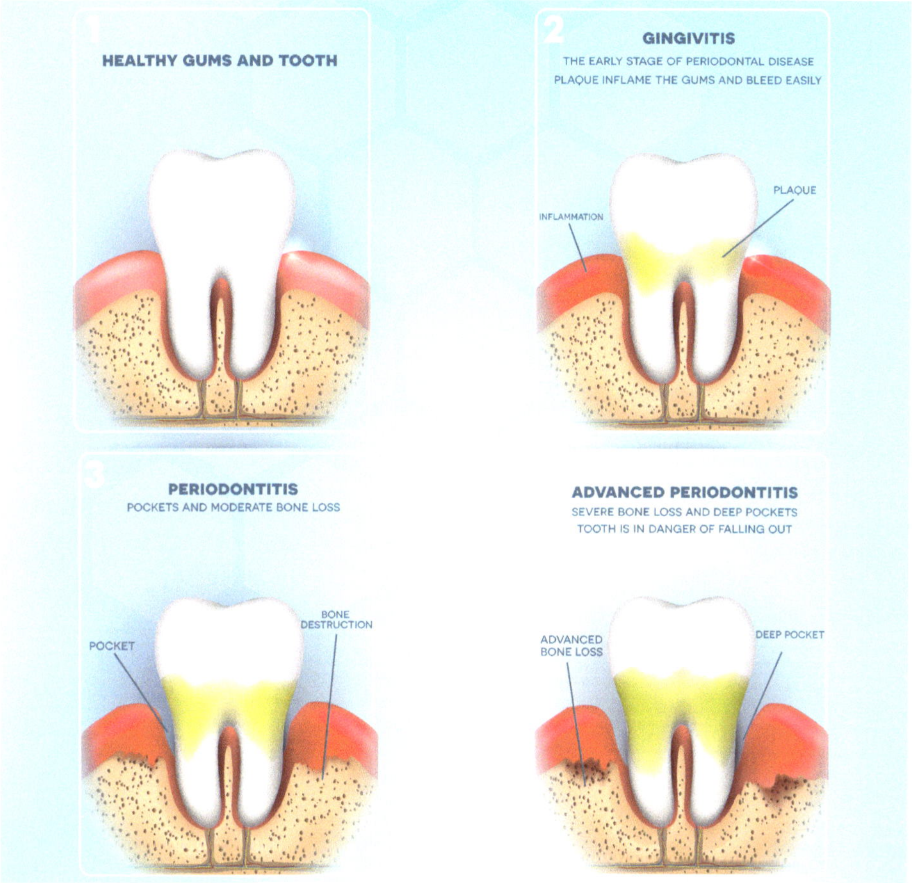

Healthy teeth = healthy body

Take care of dental problems promptly

You may be surprised to learn that ignoring a dental infection may have life-threatening consequences. If not stopped, an infection of the root canal system can spread throughout the entire body and become a systemic infection.

Take care of your dry mouth symptoms

Various medications can cause dry mouth, which may make you susceptible to dental cavities. Talk to your general dentist if you have concerns about dry mouth. There are saliva substitutes and various products on the market today that may help you with the symptoms.

Please quit smoking and chewing tobacco

Tobacco in any form has a negative impact on your oral health. It may increase the potential for dry mouth, gum disease, tooth discoloration and oral cancer.

Tooth discoloration

Endodontists are often called on to enhance the color of a tooth. Sounds odd, right? But their expertise on the internal structure of teeth makes it possible for them to improve their color from the inside out.

Discoloration, greying or darkening of a tooth may be caused by trauma. Nerve death may also cause discoloration. The by-products of the nerve and blood vessels can stain the tooth from the inside, usually over a long period of time.

Here's how endodontists improve the aesthetics of a discolored tooth. First, they complete a root canal system cleaning to eliminate the bacteria and dead nerve tissue. (This bleaching technique is always done in conjunction with a root canal system cleaning.) Second, they place a bleaching solution inside the disinfected tooth. In some cases, two bleaching treatments are needed. Third, the endodontist temporarily seals the root canal system. Fourth, the general dentist will complete the restoration with a new crown or filling.

This is another example of the ways your general dentist and endodontist work in partnership for your dental health.

About Dr. Sheila Chandrahasa

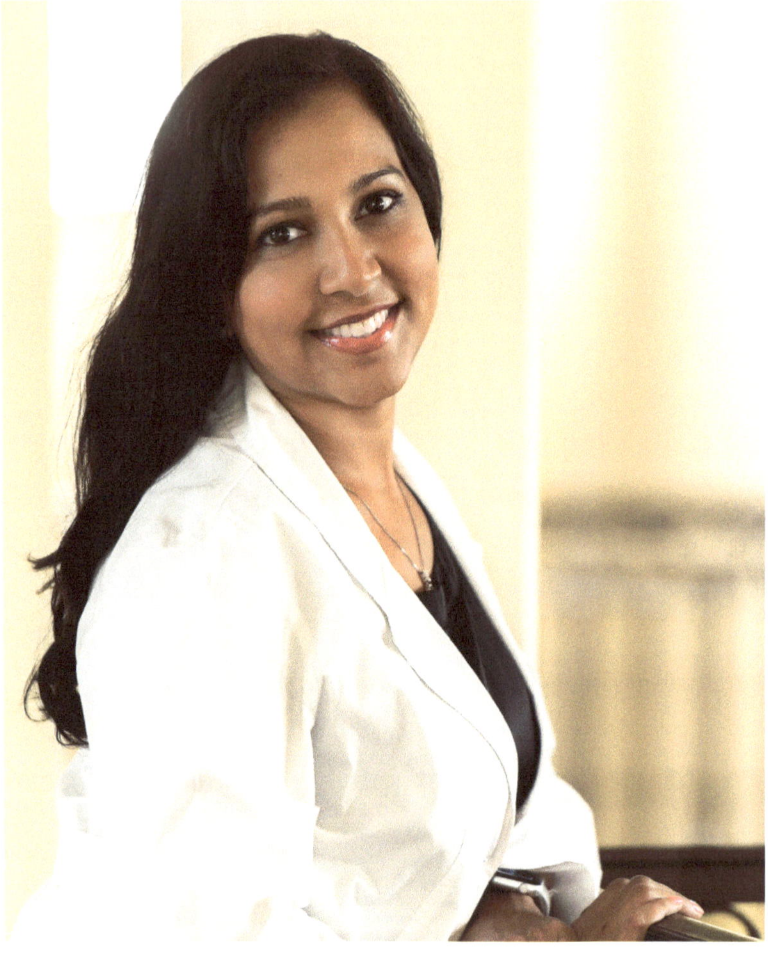

Born and raised in Port Charlotte, Florida, Dr. Chandrahasa earned her undergraduate degree in Psychology from Emory University and her Doctor of Medical Dentistry from Nova Southeastern University. She completed her General Practice Residency at the Miami Veterans Affairs Hospital and practiced as a general dentist before returning for specialty training in Endodontics.

During her Endodontics Residency, Dr. Chandrahasa conducted stem cell therapy research which was published in the *Journal of Endodontics*.

Dr. Chandrahasa treats complicated endodontic cases with care and compassion. She specializes in the diagnosis and treatment of traumatic injuries of teeth, oral pain, and both surgical and non-surgical endodontic procedures.

Dr. Chandrahasa maintains memberships in the Florida Dental Association, American Dental Association, the West Coast Dental Society and the American Association of Endodontists.

www.ingramcontent.com/pod-product-compliance
Lightning Source LLC
LaVergne TN
LVHW070626061126
851857LV00002B/20
* 9 7 8 0 5 7 8 6 2 6 0 9 3 *